Male
Reproductive System

Clinical Anatomy and Physiology

Akmal El-Mazny

ISBN-13: 978-1522888673
ISBN-10: 1522888675

CONTENTS

INTRODUCTION

The male reproductive system consists of the hypothalamic-pituitary unit, the testes, the reproductive tract, and the external genitalia.

The functions of the male reproductive system are to produce and deliver spermatozoa, for sexual reproduction, and produce hormones that regulate reproductive function and secondary sex characteristics.

Abnormalities in anatomic or physiologic function affect the development and delivery of spermatozoa, and potential fertility.

Male factors are often the cause of a couple's failure to conceive, therefore, it is important to evaluate and treat the male partner.

A male factor may be due to abnormalities of hormonal control, testicular function, or sperm transport or delivery.

This book provides a comprehensive review of the clinical anatomy and physiology specific to male reproductive system, emphasizing causes and management of male infertility.

By developing a clear understanding of what is normal, you will better understand abnormalities affecting male fertility and the mechanisms behind treatment.

OVERVIEW

<u>Basic Embryology</u>

Sex determination takes place at the time of fertilization through the coupling of two gametes, either each with one X chromosome (XX in females) or such with an X and a Y chromosome (XY in males).

Primarily, the male phenotype is determined by the presence of the Y chromosome with its genes, even though genes on other chromosomes are also involved.

In addition to the genetic factors, hormonal regulation also plays an important role during the various developmental steps.

During the first 6 weeks the genital system is sex-indifferent and it is only then that the gonads as well as the internal and external genitalia form under hormonal influence.

Two types of testicular cells are decisively important for the development of the male genitalia:

Firstly, the supporting (Sertoli) cells surround the germ cells and form the antimüllerian hormone (AMH), which causes the paramesoneophric (Müllerian) duct to atrophy.

Secondly, the interstitial (Leydig) cells produce testosterone, which is responsible for the differentiation of the male genitalia.

On both sides of the epididymis the mesonephric (Wolffian) duct forms the deferent duct, the seminal vesicle, and the ejaculatory duct and it opens into the urethra below the urinary bladder.

The urethra as well as various accessory glands (prostate, bulbourethral and urethral glands) stem from the urogenital sinus.

The penis arises from the genital tubercle and the urethral folds and the scrotum from the genital swellings.

Sexual Differentation

Basic Anatomy and Physiology

The male reproductive system is a network of external and internal organs.

Male gonads are the testes, which produce sperm (exocrine function) and hormones (endocrine function).

Sperm produced in the testes is transported through the epididymis, ductus deferens, ejaculatory duct, and urethra.

The seminal vesicles, prostate gland, and bulbourethral gland produce seminal fluid that accompany and nourish the sperm as it is emitted from the penis during ejaculation and throughout the fertilization process.

Male Reproductive System

Male Infertility

Infertility is defined by the World Health Organization (WHO) as the absence of conception after at least 12 months of unprotected intercourse.

An estimated 10-15% of couples meets this criterion and are considered infertile.

Isolated conditions of the female are responsible for infertility in 35% of cases, isolated conditions of the male in 30%, conditions of both the male and female in 20%, and unexplained causes in 15%.

A male factor may be due to hormonal abnormalities resulting in decreased sperm production, abnormalities of testicular function or abnormal sperm transport or delivery.

The initial evaluation of the male patient should be rapid, noninvasive, and cost-effective, as nearly 70% of conditions that cause infertility in men can be diagnosed with history, physical examination, and hormonal and semen analysis alone.

More detailed, invasive, and expensive studies can then be ordered if necessary.

Treatment options are based on the underlying etiology and range from optimizing semen production and transportation with medical therapy or surgical procedures to complex assisted reproduction techniques.

HORMONAL CONTROL

Several hormones control testes function:

−GnRH is secreted by the hypothalamus and stimulates the pituitary to synthesize and release LH and FSH.

−LH stimulates Leydig cells to synthesize testosterone.

−FSH maintains Sertoli cell function.

Effects of Testosterone

Testosterone has significant reproductive and nonreproductive effects throughout the male life cycle.

Before birth, testosterone masculinizes the reproductive tract and external genitalia and promotes descent of the testes into the scrotum.

For sex-specific tissues, testosterone promotes growth and maturation of the reproductive system at puberty, is essential for spermatogenesis, and maintains the reproductive tract throughout adulthood.

Other reproductive effects include development of the sex drive at puberty and control of gonadotropin hormone secretion; secondary sex characteristics are also testosterone-dependent.

Testosterone induces the male pattern of hair growth (such as the beard), causes the voice to deepen due to thickening of the vocal cords, and promotes muscle growth responsible for the male body configuration.

Nonreproductive actions of testosterone include a protein anabolic effect, promotion of bone growth at puberty and closure of the epiphyseal plates.

Pituitary Feedback

Testosterone provides negative feedback to the pituitary to decrease LH and FSH levels, and to the hypothalamus to decrease GnRH production.

Inhibin, produced by Sertoli cells, is responsible for the remainder of the inhibition of FSH production.

Hormonal Control of Testicular Function

PRETESTICULAR CAUSES OF INFERTILITY

Pretesticular causes of infertility include congenital or acquired diseases of the hypothalamus, pituitary, or peripheral organs that alter the hypothalamic-pituitary axis.

Disorders of the hypothalamus lead to hypogonadotropic hypogonadism.

If GnRH is not secreted, the pituitary does not release LH and FSH.

Ideally, patients respond to replacement with exogenous GnRH or HCG, an LH analogue, although this does not always occur.

Kallmann Syndrome

Kallmann syndrome patients lack GnRH production and lack the nerves enabling their sense of smell, called anosmia.

Patients with GnRH deficiency do not produce LH and FSH, with resulting azoospermia.

Gonadotropin replacement therapy can reverse the azoospermia.

Abnormalities associated with Kallmann syndrome include anosmia, cryptorchidism, and gynecomastia.

Prader-Willi Syndrome

Prader-Willi Syndrome is a complex genetic condition that involves the loss of genes in a specific region of chromosome 15.

It results in low levels of FSH and LH, hypotonia, obesity, mental retardation, and short stature.

Laurence-Moon-Biedl Syndrome

Laurence-Moon-Biedl syndrome or Laurence-Moon syndrome is a rare inherited disorder characterized by diminished hormone production by the testes (hypogonadism).

Affected individuals have microphallus, hypospadias, undescended testes, and obesity.

Prolactinoma

A prolactin-secreting adenoma is the most common functional pituitary tumor.

Prolactin stimulates breast development and lactation; therefore, patients with infertility due to a prolactinoma may have gynecomastia and galactorrhea.

In addition, loss of peripheral visual fields bilaterally may be due to compression of the optic chiasm by the growing pituitary tumor.

A prolactin level of more than 150 mcg/L suggests a pituitary adenoma.

Levels greater than 300 mcg/L are nearly diagnostic.

Patients should undergo an MRI or CT scan of the sella turcica for diagnostic purposes to determine whether a microprolactinoma or a macroprolactinoma is present.

Bromocriptine and cabergoline are dopamine agonists used to suppress prolactin levels.

These are both treatment options for microprolactinoma.

Some men respond with an increase in testosterone levels; many also recover normal sperm counts.

Transsphenoidal resection of a microprolactinoma is 80-90% successful, but as many as 17% recur.

Surgical therapy of a macroprolactinoma is rarely curative, although this should be considered in patients with visual-field defects or those who do not tolerate bromocriptine.

Isolated LH Deficiency

Isolated LH deficiency is also known as "fertile eunuch syndrome."

This is a variant of Kallmann syndrome where enough FSH is produced to induce spermatogenesis despite incomplete sexual development.

Isolated FSH Deficiency

This is a very rare cause of infertility.

Patients present with oligospermia but have normal LH levels.

Treatment is with HMG or exogenous FSH.

Thalassemia

Patients with thalassemia have ineffective erythropoiesis and undergo multiple blood transfusions.

Excess iron from multiple transfusions may get deposited in the pituitary gland and the testis, causing parenchymal damage.

Treatment is with exogenous gonadotropins and iron-chelating therapy.

Cushing Disease

Increased cortisol levels cause a negative feedback on the hypothalamus, decreasing GnRH release.

Congenital Adrenal Hyperplasia (CAH)

CAH may be due to the congenital deficiency of one of several adrenal enzymes, the most common of which is 21-hydroxylase deficiency.

Because cortisol is not secreted, a lack of feedback inhibition on the pituitary gland occurs, leading to ACTH hypersecretion.

This leads to increased androgen secretion from the adrenal gland, causing feedback inhibition of GnRH release from the hypothalamus.

Patients present with short stature, precocious puberty, small testis, and occasional bilateral testicular rests.

Screening tests include increased plasma 17-hydroxylase and urine 17-ketosteroids.

Estrogen Excess

Estrogen excess, in patients with Sertoli cell tumors, Leydig tumors, liver failure, or severe obesity, causes negative feedback on the pituitary gland, inhibiting LH and FSH release.

TESTES

The testes are the primary male reproductive organ and are responsible for testosterone and sperm production.

Their development is influenced by the presence of the Y sex chromosome and by maternal hormonal levels.

The testes develop in the fetal abdomen and begin descent during the 7th month of pregnancy.

The male sex organs are formed under the influence of testosterone secreted from the fetal testes.

Failure to descend, called cryptorchidism, results in sterility, which is a lack of spermatozoa, and, frequently, abnormally low testosterone.

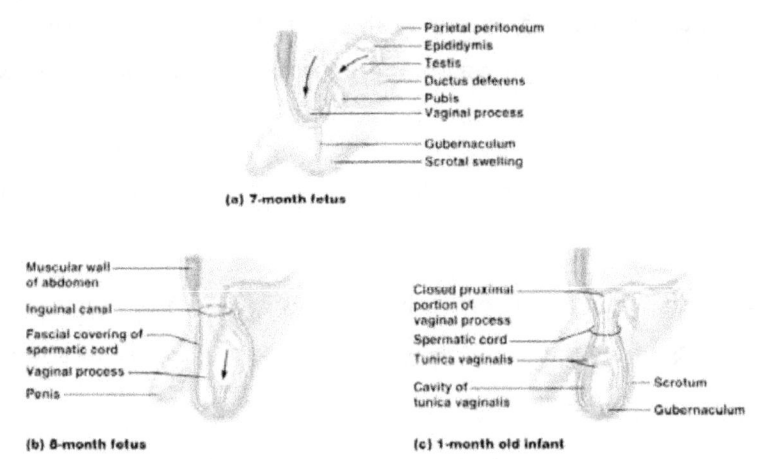

Testicular Descend

Each testis is 4-5 cm long, 2-3 cm wide, weighs 10-14 g and is suspended in the scrotum by the dartos muscle and spermatic cord.

Suspension outside the body cavity permits spermatogenesis at 36°C.

Each testis is covered by the tunica vaginalis testis, tunica albuginea, and tunica vasculosa.

The tunica vaginalis testis is the lower portion of the processus vaginalis and is reflected from the testes on the inner surface of the scrotum, thus forming the visceral and parietal layers.

Beneath the visceral layer of the tunica vaginalis is the tunica albuginea, which forms a dense covering for the testes.

Internal to the tunica albuginea is the tunica vasculosa, containing a plexus of blood vessels and connective tissue.

Bilateral testicular arteries originating from the aorta, just inferior to the renal arteries, enter the scrotum in the spermatic cord via the inguinal canal, and split into two branches at the posterosuperior border of the testis.

Additionally, the testes receive blood from the cremasteric branch of the inferior epigastric artery and the artery to the ductus deferens.

The pampiniform plexus drains both the testis and epididymis before coalescing to form the testicular vein, usually above the spermatic cord formation at the deep inguinal ring.

Lymphatic drainage via the testicular vessels passes into the abdomen, ending in the lateral aortic and pre-aortic nodes.

The tenth and eleventh thoracic spinal nerves supply the testes via the renal and aortic autonomic plexuses.

Scrotum

The scrotum is a fibromuscular pouch divided by a median septum (raphe) forming 2 compartments, each of which contains a testis, epididymis and part of the spermatic cord.

Layers of the scrotum consist of skin, dartos muscle, external spermatic fascia, cremasteric fascia and internal spermatic fascia, which is in close contact with the parietal layer of the tunica vaginalis.

The skin and dartos layers of the scrotum are supplied by the perineal branch of the internal pudendal artery in addition to the external pudendal branches of the femoral artery.

The layers deep to the dartos muscle are supplied by the cremasteric branch of the inferior epigastric artery.

The veins of the scrotum accompany the arteries, eventually draining into the external pudendal vein and subsequently into the greater saphenous vein.

Lymphatic drainage of the skin of the scrotum is by the external pudendal vessels to the medial superficial inguinal lymph nodes .

The scrotum has a rich sensory nerve supply that includes the genital branch of the genitofemoral nerve (anterior and lateral scrotal surfaces), the ilioinguinal nerve (anterior scrotal surface), posterior scrotal branches of the perineal nerve (posterior scrotal surface), and the perineal branch of the posterior femoral cutaneous nerve (inferior scrotal surface).

Microscopic Anatomy

The testes are divided into approximately 400 segments called lobules each of which is occupied by 2-4 seminiferous tubules, which are responsible for producing spermatozoa.

Each testis has 600-1200 seminiferous tubules with a total length of 280-400-m.

At the mediastinum testis, on the posterior border of the testis, the seminiferous tubules empty spermatozoa into the tubuli recti and rete testis, eventually coalescing to form 6-8 efferent ductules draining spermatozoa into the epididymis.

The seminiferous tubule epithelium consists of proliferating spermatogenic cells and the sustentacular Sertoli cells.

Spermatogenic cells are at various stages of spermatogenesis and Sertoli cells are columnar cells that extend from the basement membrane to the lumen of the seminiferous tubule.

Interstitial cells in the testis, including the Leydig cells, constitute 20-30% of the tissue in the gland and are found in between seminiferous tubules.

The washed out cytoplasm of the Leydig cells is due high lipid content in the form of cholesterol for synthesis of testosterone.

Seminiferous Tubules

The seminiferous tubules are the site of spermatogenesis; there are approximately 244 m (800 feet) of seminiferous tubules in each testis.

Each tubule consists of a basement membrane, lined with germ cells that become spermatozoa, and Sertoli cells; these tubules increase in diameter and tortuosity with hormonal changes of puberty.

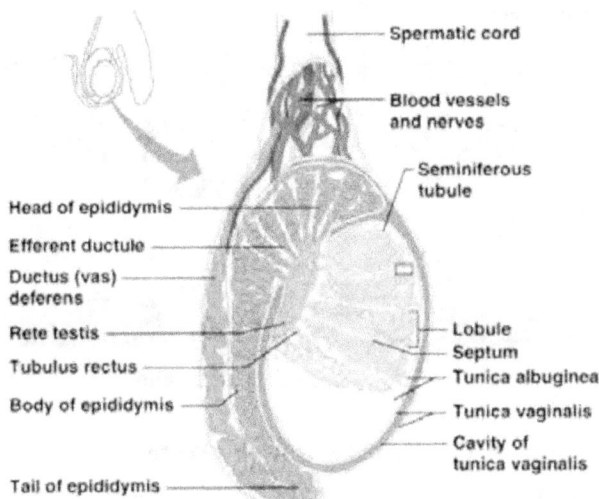

Seminiferous Tubules

Cell Types within the Testes

There are three unique cell types within the testes:

– Germ cells, the cells that divide and mature to become sperm.

– Sertoli cells, which provide crucial support for spermatogenesis.

– Leydig cells that produce the androgenic hormone testosterone, which maintains the reproductive tract and secondary sex characteristics.

All germ cells and Sertoli cells are within the seminiferous tubule, while Leydig cells are outside the tubules.

Cell Types within the Testes

Sertoli Cells

The Sertoli cells of the testes are joined together by tight junctions that form the blood-testis barrier, which prevents diffusion of plasma constituents into the tubular lumen.

The blood-testis barrier also prevents contact between germ cells and blood, which is important because spermatozoa are antigenic.

Sertoli cells nourish developing sperm, and have a phagocytic function to destroy defective germ cells and engulf extruded cytoplasm from spermatids during remodeling.

Sertoli cells secrete seminiferous tubule fluid, androgen-binding protein and inhibin and activin, which regulate FSH secretion.

Leydig Cells

Interstitial cells in the testis, including the Leydig cells, constitute 20-30% of the tissue in the gland and are found in between seminiferous tubules.

The washed out cytoplasm of the Leydig cells is due high lipid content in the form of cholesterol for synthesis of testosterone.

The interstitial Leydig cells produce and secrete testosterone which is absolutely required for spermatogenesis.

However, FSH greatly enhances spermatogenesis by stimulating the functions of Sertoli cells and increasing mitoses of spermatogonia.

Once mitosis has been initiated in spermatogonia, testosterone alone can maintain spermatogenesis.

Functions

– Produce germ cells (spermatozoa) for sexual reproduction.

– Produce testosterone that regulates reproductive function and secondary sex characteristics.

SPERMATOGENESIS

Beginning at puberty, spermatogenesis occurs continuously and repeatedly within folds of the Sertoli cells.

Spermatogonia (the sperm stem cells) lie at the base of the Sertoli cells and proliferate through mitosis to produce daughter cells that enter spermatogenesis.

In the two-step reduction division process of meiosis, spermatocytes and spermatids develop; spermatids are haploid, containing only one copy of each chromosome.

As the germ cells divide and mature, they move away from the base of the tubule toward the apical surface of Sertoli cells.

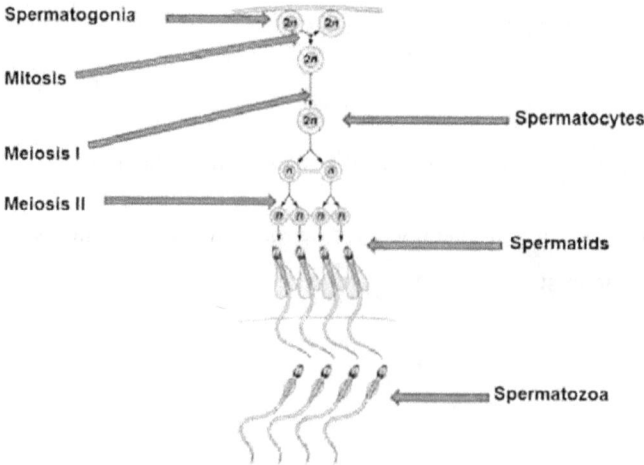

Spermatogenesis

Spermiogenesis

Following meiosis, spermiogenesis is the maturation process in which the round spermatids are transformed into elongated spermatozoa with tails.

The spermatid nucleus condenses and most cytoplasm is lost; the Golgi apparatus moves to one side of the nucleus, forming an acrosome that surrounds the top two thirds of the nucleus (in the head).

Cell microtubules organize into a flagellar apparatus to form the tail for motility, and mitochondria for movement.

Spermiogenesis

Spermiation

Spermiation is the process in which fully developed but non-motile spermatozoa are released from the Sertoli cells and propelled out of the tubules into the collecting tubules, rete testis and then the epididymis.

Spermiation

Mature Sperm

Mature sperm have a head, which consists primarily of the nucleus containing genetic information.

The acrosome is a specialized lysosome, containing about 20 different enzymes, which are needed for penetration of the ovum during fertilization.

The acrosome covers the anterior third of the nucleus in a mature sperm.

In the midpiece are mitochondria to provide the energy required for the movement of the tail.

The tail grows out of one of the centrioles; movement results from the sliding of the microtubules.

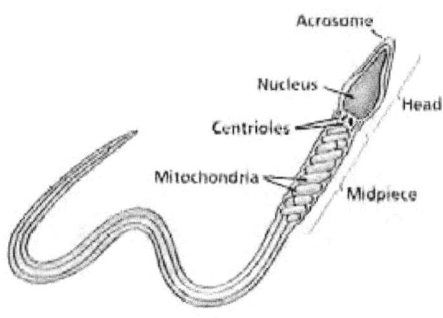

Mature Sperm

Normal Sperm Morphology

Normal sperm morphology is defined by multiple parameters:

- The head is oval shaped, 4-5 microns long, 2-3 microns wide, the length-to-width ratio is 1.5 to 1.75, and a well-defined acrosome makes up 40 to 70% of the head area.

- The midpiece is intact and there is no cytoplasmic droplet.

- The tail is 45 microns long, and is not bent or coiled.

Sperm Abnormalities

Sperm abnormalities are scored in four categories:

- For the head, abnormal characteristics include large, small, tapered, pyriform, amorphous, vacuolated, bicephalic, and acrosome defects.

- In the neck and midpiece, a distended or irregular midpiece, thin midpiece (no mitochondria), and bent or absent tail are abnormal.

- Abnormal tails may be short, multiple, hairpin, broken, or coiled.

- If there is a cytoplasmic droplet attached at the midpiece, the spermatozoon is considered immature.

Manual Assessment of Sperm Motility

Qualitative evaluation of forward motion:

0 = immotile.

1 = tail movement with no forward movement of the sperm.

2 = weak forward progression.

3 = active tail movement with good forward progression.

4 = vigorous tail movement with rapid forward progression.

TESTICULAR CAUSES OF INFERTILITY

Primary testicular problems may be chromosomal or nonchromosomal.

While chromosomal failure is usually caused by abnormalities of the sex chromosomes, autosomal disorders are also observed.

Chromosomal Abnormalities

An estimated 6-13% of infertile men have chromosomal abnormalities (compared with 0.6% of the general population).

Patients with azoospermia or severe oligospermia are more likely to have a chromosomal abnormality (10-15%) than infertile men with sperm density within the reference range (1%).

Klinefelter Syndrome (47, XXY)

The most common sex chromosome disorder is Klinefelter syndrome, which is due to the presence of an extra X chromosome (47, XXY) and occurs in about 1 out of every 1000 males.

Men with Klinefelter syndrome have high FSH levels and may have low testosterone levels.

They characteristically have small, firm testes and azoospermia.

While some men have bilateral gynecomastia (breast enlargement), delayed puberty and a female body shape with relatively long legs, many men appear normal but only have small testes and infertility.

Some men have a mosaic pattern on karyotype (47, XXY/46, XY) and may have oligospermia.

XX Male

The 46, XX male is rare.

Although the karyotype is female, individuals are phenotypically males, with male external genitalia ranging from normal to ambiguous; two testicles; azoospermia; and absence of müllerian structures.

XYY Male

An XYY karyotype is observed in 0.1-0.4% of newborn males.

These patients are often tall and severely oligospermic or azoospermic.

This pattern has been linked with aggressive behavior.

Biopsy reveals maturation arrest or germ cell aplasia.

Noonan Syndrome

Noonan syndrome is sometimes referred to as male Turner syndrome and has autosomal dominant inheritance.

Defects in four genes (KRAS, PTPN11, RAF1, SOS1) affect proteins involved in the proper formation of several types of tissue during development, including sexual organs.

Individuals with Noonan syndrome typically have unusual facial characteristics, short stature, heart defects, bleeding problems, skeletal malformations and eye abnormalities.

Most with Noonan syndrome have normal intelligence, but puberty is usually delayed and most males have undescended testicles and diminished spermatogenesis.

Mixed Gonadal Dysgenesis (45, X/46, XY)

Patients have ambiguous genitalia, a testis on one side, and a streaked gonad on the other.

Y-chromosome Microdeletions

Y-chromosome microdeletions are found in 10 to 15% of men with azoospermia and severe oligospermia.

This condition involves the long arm (Yq11) of the Y chromosome.

There are 3 regions: Azoospermia Factor AZFa, AZFb, AZFc.

Deletion of the entire AZFa or AZFb region results in azoospermia.

Men with AZFc deletions may have azoospermia or oligospermia.

Bilateral Anorchia (Vanishing Testis Syndrome)

Patients have a normal male karyotype (46, XY) and phenotype but are born without testis.

Potential causes are unknown, but it may be related to infection, vascular disease, or bilateral testicular torsion.

Patients may achieve normal virilization and adult phenotype by the administration of exogenous testosterone, but they are infertile.

Down Syndrome

These patients have mild testicular dysfunction with varying degrees of reduction in germ cell number.

LH and FSH levels are usually elevated.

Myotonic Muscular Dystrophy

Myotonic muscular dystrophy is an inherited disorder of progressive muscle degeneration.

It has an autosomal dominant pattern involving chromosome 19 and is the most common form of muscular dystrophy that begins in adulthood.

The condition causes hypergonadotropic hypogonadism, with elevated FSH and LH with low testosterone.

These men experience atrophy of the testicles and reduced fertility.

Congenital Deficiency of Testosterone Production

Congenital deficiency of testosterone production is a rare disorder that is caused by a lack of genes that encode for androgen enzymes biosynthesis.

There is incomplete virilization in affected men.

Nonchromosomal Testicular Failure

Testicular failure that is nonchromosomal in origin may be idiopathic or acquired by gonadotoxic drugs, radiation, orchitis, trauma, or torsion.

Varicocele

This is the most common correctable cause of male infertility.

Varicocele is present in 15% of all males and in 40% of infertile males.

A varicocele is an abnormal dilation of the veins of the pampiniform plexus in the scrotum; usually left-sided, but may be bilateral.

Varicoceles have a progressive deleterious effect on spermatogenesis.

Cryptorchidism

There is a failure of the testes to descend into the scrotum.

It is the most common birth defect of the male genitalia.

In boys born at full term, the cause is usually unknown.

About 30% of men with unilateral cryptorchidism and 50% of men with bilateral cryptorchidism will have oligospermia.

Androgen Insensitivity Syndrome (AIS)

Androgen insensitivity syndrome, or AIS, was formerly known as "testicular feminization".

In this condition, there is a defect in the androgen receptor gene, which results in a lack of androgen receptors, a defect in receptor function, or post-receptor defects.

Individuals with androgen insensitivity syndrome are genetic males (46, XY) but have a female phenotype.

Testes are undescended, there is a lack of pubic hair, and the proximal vagina, uterus and tubes are absent.

The condition affects 2 to 5 per 100,000 people who are genetically male.

Trauma

Testicular trauma is the second most common acquired infertility.

The testes are at risk for both thermal and physical trauma because of their exposed position.

Sertoli-cell-only Syndrome

Developmental abnormalities include Sertoli-cell-only syndrome, also known as germ cell aplasia.

In this condition, there is congenital absence of germ cells in the seminiferous tubules of the testes due to failure of migration during embryonic development.

As a result, only Sertoli cells line the seminiferous tubules of the testes.

A pattern of Sertoli-cell-only can also be acquired as a result of exposure to chemotherapy or radiation therapy that destroys the germ cells.

Some men have small pockets of sperm production within portions of the testicle, which can be retrieved by testicular sperm extraction.

Chemotherapy

Chemotherapy is toxic to actively dividing cells.

In the testicle, germ cells (especially up to the preleptotene stage) are especially at risk.

The agents most often associated with infertility are the alkylating agents such as cyclophosphamide.

For example, treatment for Hodgkin disease has been estimated to lead to infertility in as many as 80-100% of patients.

Radiation Therapy

While Leydig cells are relatively radioresistant because of their low rate of cell division, the Sertoli and germ cells are extremely radiosensitive.

If stem cells remain viable after radiation therapy, patients may regain fertility within several years.

However, some have suggested that patients should avoid conception for 6 months to 2 years after completion of radiation therapy because of the possibility of chromosomal aberrations in their sperm caused by the mutagenic properties of radiation therapy.

Orchitis

The most common cause of acquired testicular failure in adults is viral orchitis, such as mumps virus, echovirus, or group B arbovirus.

The virus may either directly damage the seminiferous tubules or indirectly cause ischemic damage as the intense swelling leads to compression against the tough tunica albuginea.

Normal fertility is observed in three fourths of patients with unilateral mumps orchitis and in one third of patients in bilateral orchitis.

Idiopathic Causes

Despite a thorough workup, nearly 25% of men have no discernible cause for their infertility.

DUCT SYSTEM

For each testis there is a duct system; the function of these ducts is testosterone-dependent.

The cells absorb fluid from the testis and remove particulate matter by endocytosis.

The epididymis is where sperm mature, concentrate and are stored for five to six days in this segment of the tract.

The vas deferens is a secondary storage site for spermatozoa; its epithelium has important absorptive and secretory functions.

The other components of the duct system are the ejaculatory duct and the urethra.

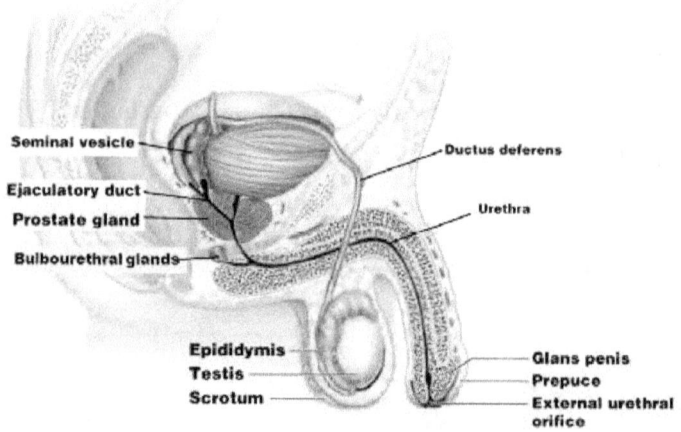

Duct System

Epididymis

The epididymis is a C-shaped structure lying intimately along the posterior border of each testis.

It includes an enlarged head, a body and a tail.

The tunica vaginalis covers the epididymis except at the posterior border.

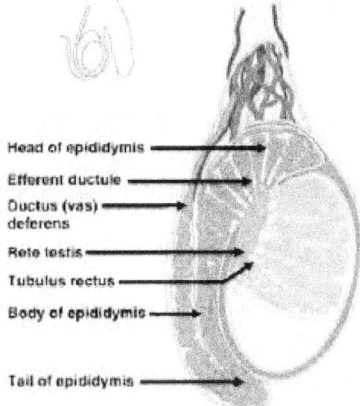

Head of epididymis
Efferent ductule
Ductus (vas) deferens
Rete testis
Tubulus rectus
Body of epididymis
Tail of epididymis

Epididymis

Vasculature and innervation of the epididymis is the same as for the testes.

Microscopic Anatomy

The main component of the epididymis is a tightly packed, tortuous duct approximately 6-m long and 400-μm in diameter.

The head consists of the most dense pack coils of efferent ductules, which are lined with ciliated columnar epithelium for transport of spermatozoa through the epididymis.

Functions

The epididymis is the major storage site of spermatozoa, which spend five to six days in this segment of the tract.

When sperm initially enter the epididymis, they are immotile and do not have the capacity to fertilize ova.

Tight junctions between epididymal epithelial cells maintain the blood-testis barrier, which is important for immune protection of sperm.

Epididymal fluid is enriched in potassium relative to semen and rich in glycerophosphorylcholine, a major energy source for spermatozoa .

The epididymis responds preferentially to dihydrotestosterone.

The epididymal histology and function change along its length:

– The initial segment connects with the rete testis and has tall columnar cells and a narrow lumen for major fluid absorption.

– In the caput, fluid becomes hyperosmotic and sperm attain motility.

– In the corpus, fertilizing potential is achieved with maturation of the sperm plasma membrane and sperm attain the ability to adhere to the zona pellucida of the ovum.

– In the cauda are cuboidal cells with a wide lumen for sperm storage; the luminal fluid becomes acidic as it moves from caput to cauda.

Ductus (Vas) Deferens

The ductus (vas) deferens is the continuation of the epididymis; it is 30-45-cm long and conveys sperm to the ejaculatory ducts.

The convoluted portion of ductus deferens becomes straighter (diameter, 2-3-mm) as it travels posterior to the testis and medial to the epididymis.

Subsequently, the ductus ascends on the posterior aspect of the spermatic cord until it reaches the deep inguinal ring, where it participates in the formation of spermatic cord and loops over the inferior epigastric artery.

At this point, the ductus travels along the lateral pelvic wall, medial to the distal ureter, along the posterior wall of the bladder until it reaches the seminal vesicles dorsal to the prostate.

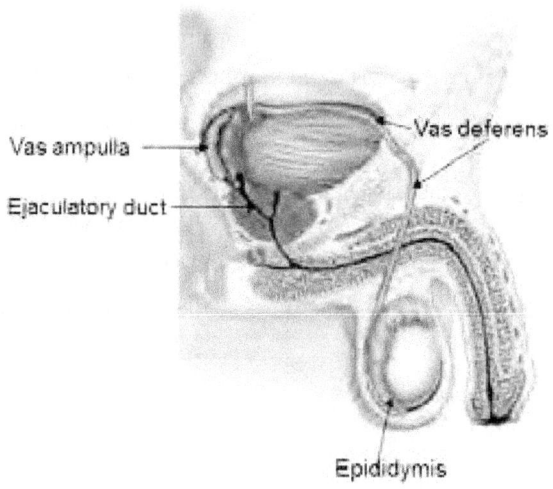

Ductus (Vas) Deferens

Each ductus deferens has an artery usually derived from the superior vesical artery (artery to the ductus).

Venous drainage is to the pelvic venous plexus.

Lymphatic drainage is to the external and internal iliac nodes.

Innervation is mainly sympathetic from the pelvic plexus.

Microscopic Anatomy

The ductus deferens is composed of pseudostratified columnar epithelium including columnar cells and basal cells.

The underlying lamina propria is dense with elastic fibers and the wall of the ductus contains three thick smooth muscle layers.

The outermost layer of adventitia is rich in blood vessels and nerves.

Functions

In the ductus deferens, there is rapid transport of sperm during ejaculation and slow transport and removal of excess sperm during sexual rest.

The proximal part of the vas is the site of vasectomy for contraception.

The distal part near the prostate, called the ampulla, stores sperm and empties into ejaculatory ducts that traverse the prostate gland to enter the urethra.

Spermatic Cord

The spermatic cord extends from the deep inguinal ring, through the inguinal canal to the testis.

The layers of the spermatic cord include (from outward to inward):

– External spermatic fascia (derived from the deep fascia of the external abdominal oblique muscle).

– Cremasteric fascia (derived from the internal oblique muscle).

– Internal spermatic fascia (derived from the transversalis fascia).

The structures that form the spermatic cord include:

– The ductus deferens and associated vasculature and nerves (posterior wall of the cord).

– The testicular artery.

– The pampiniform plexus, ultimately forming the testicular vein.

– The genital branch of the genitofemoral nerve.

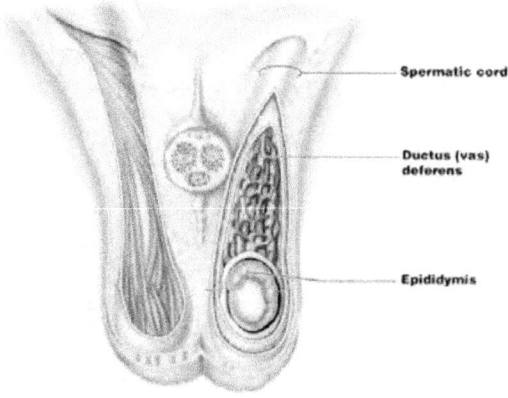

Spermatic cord

Ejaculatory Ducts

The ejaculatory ducts are 2-cm in length and derived from the union of the seminal vesicle and the ampulla of the vas deferens.

Each duct starts at the base of the prostate and terminates at the seminal colliculus (verumontanum).

The vasculature, innervation, and lymphatics of the ejaculatory ducts are the same as for the ductus deferens.

Urethra

The urethra stretches from the bladder to the tip of the glans penis, serving as a passage for urine and semen.

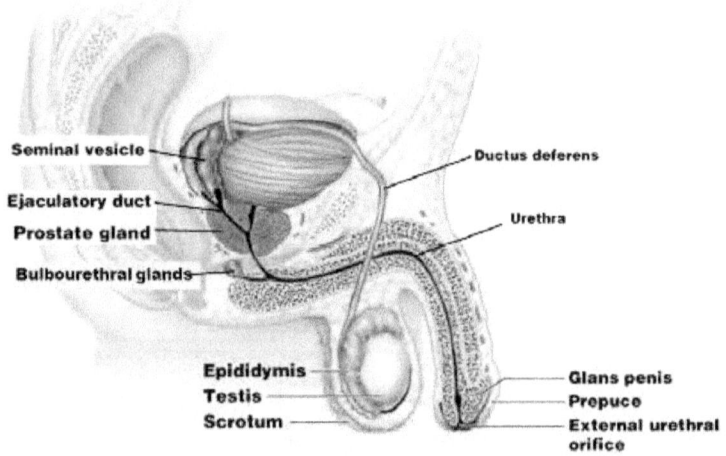

Male Urethra

The prostatic urethra extends vertically from the bladder neck, through the prostate before becoming the membranous urethra and before penetrating the perineal membrane; of note, the prostatic urethra contains the orifice of the ejaculatory ducts.

As the membranous urethra enters the deep perineal space, the urethra is surrounded by fibers of the external urethral sphincter, eventually entering the bulb of the corpus spongiosum, providing the orifice for the bulbourethral glands and subsequently becoming the penile urethra.

When the urethra reaches the glans penis the diameter diminishes to that of the external ostium, the least dilatable portion of the urethral canal.

Microscopic Anatomy

– The prostatic urethra is lined by transitional epithelium,

– The membranous urethra is lined by stratified columnar epithelium, and

– The penile urethra is initially stratified columnar epithelium and becomes stratified squamous epithelium at the fossa navicularis.

ACCESSORY GLANDS

Accessory glands include the seminal vesicle, prostate gland and bulbourethral glands.

The seminal vesicle provides precursor proteins responsible for semen coagulation, supplies fructose to nourish the ejaculated sperm and secretes prostaglandins that stimulate motility.

The prostate gland secretes proteolytic enzymes to liquefy coagulum after ejaculation, alkaline fluid to neutralize acidic vaginal secretions and the high zinc content is antimicrobial.

The bulbourethral glands, also known as Cowper's glands, secrete mucus for lubrication.

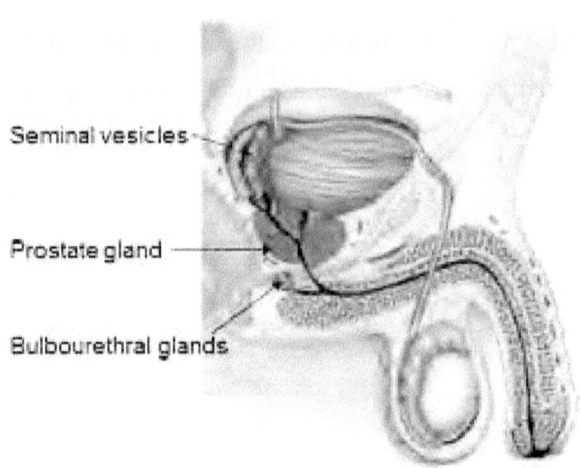

Accessory Glands

Seminal Vesicles

The 2 seminal vesicles are located between the bladder and the rectum and measure approximately 5 cm in length.

The anterior surface is in contact with the posterior wall of the bladder and the posterior surface is in contact with rectovesical fascia.

The ampulla of the ductus deferens lies medial to the seminal vesicles and the prostatic venous plexus lies laterally.

Arterial blood supply to the seminal vesicles includes branches from the inferior vesical and middle rectal arteries, while venous and lymphatic drainage accompanies these arteries.

The inferior division of the hypogastric plexus provides innervation to the seminal vesicles.

Microscopic Anatomy

The seminal vesicles are tubulosaccular glands consisting of connective tissue and secretory epithelium projecting into the lumen of the gland.

The epithelium is pseudostratified with basal and columnar cells, while the wall of the vesicle is consistent with a thick wall of smooth muscle.

Functions

The seminal vesicles, which are testosterone-dependent, have important secretory function, but they have little storage capacity.

They produce a very alkaline secretion and fibrin, which is responsible for coagulation of semen after ejaculation.

Prostate

The prostate gland is an ovoid structure encompassing the proximal portion of the urethra and

It is approximately 2.5-3.0 cm by 4.0-4.5 cm, and normally weighing 20-25 g.

Relations of the prostate gland:

– The base of the prostate is in contact with the bladder.

– The apex is superior to the perineal membrane.

– The anterior border is in contact with the vesicoprostatic plexus.

– The posterior border is separated from the anterior surface of the rectum by the rectovesical (Denonvilliers) fascia.

– The lateral border is in contact with the levator ani and the prostatic venous plexus.

– Fibers of the external urethral sphincter surround the prostate.

The arterial supply to the prostate gland is derived from the inferior vesical artery and branches of the middle rectal artery.

Venous drainage of the prostate forms the prostatic plexus, which eventually drains into the internal iliac vein.

Lymphatic drainage flows to the internal iliac nodes.

Innervation is derived from the inferior portion of the hypogastric plexus, primarily to the connective tissue surrounding the gland.

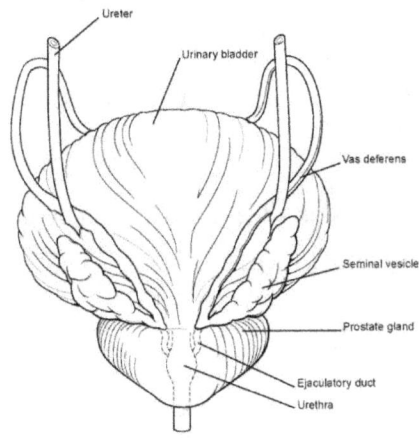

Labels: Ureter, Urinary bladder, Vas deferens, Seminal vesicle, Prostate gland, Ejaculatory duct, Urethra

Prostate Gland

Microscopic Anatomy

The prostate is traditionally divided into three concentric zones:

– The peripheral zone constitutes 70% of the prostate and contains the tubuloalveolar glands of the organ.

– The central zone constitutes 25% and contains submucosal glands.

– The transitional zone constitutes 5% of the prostate.

The tubuloalveolar glands are embedded in a fibrous stroma and open through branching ducts in the prostatic urethra.

The secretory nature of the epithelium is evident as it consists of pseudostratified epithelium containing basal and secretory cells.

Functions

The prostate gland, which is dihydrotestosterone-dependent, produces a slightly acidic (pH 6.5), colorless, thin secretion, rich in minerals and sodium.

The prostate gland produces the enzyme fibrinolysin, which degrades the fibrin clot in coagulated semen.

Bulbourethral Glands

The bilateral bulbourethral glands are 2 cm in diameter and lie lateral to the membranous urethra and are enclosed by the external urethral sphincter.

The excretory duct of the gland penetrates the perineal membrane and opens within the bulbar urethra.

Vasculature, lymphatic drainage, and innervation are generally the same as for the seminal vesicles.

The bulbourethral glands secrete mucus for lubrication during sexual intercourse.

PENIS

The penis is made up of an attached root and a pendulous body.

The root consists of two crura and the bulb - 3 bodies of erectile tissue attached to the pubic arch (crura) and perineal membrane (bulb).

Near the border of the pubic sypmphysis the bilateral crura continue as the corpora cavernosa throughout the body of the penis.

The bulb lies between the two crura, narrows anteriorly and continues as the corpus spongiosum.

The corpora cavernosa are enveloped in a thick fibrous tunica albuginea, which is comprised of a longitudinal running superficial fibers and a deep layer of circular oriented fibers.

The corpus spongiosum is penetrated by the urethra as it traverses the body of the penis.

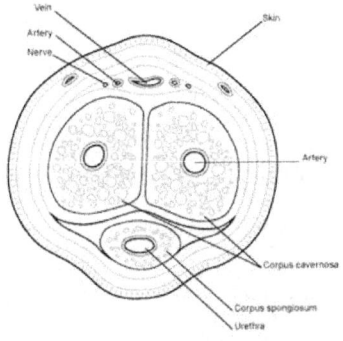

Cross-sectional Anatomy of the Penis

The superficial penile fascia includes loose connective tissue intertwined with dartos muscle fibers.

The deep penile fascia, or Buck's fascia, is a tough fascial layer that encompasses both corpora cavernosa and the corporus spongiosum.

The skin of the penis is thin; the corona of the penis is where the skin folds to become the prepuce (foreskin), enveloping the glans penis.

The vasculature of the penis is extensive.

The perineal artery (a branch of the internal pudendal artery) together with the posterior scrotal artery and the inferior rectal artery supply tissues from the bulb of the penis to the anus.

The artery of the bulb of the penis, from the internal pudendal, penetrates the penile bulb and subsequently supplies the corpus spongiosum.

The deep artery of the penis, one of two terminal branches of the internal pudendal artery, enters the crus of the penis and continues through the length of the bilateral corpus cavernosum.

The other terminal branch of the internal pudendal artery is the dorsal artery of the penis running along the dorsal surface of the penis supplying the penile skin and the glans penis.

The venous drainage of the penis includes the veins draining the corpora cavernosa, which subsequently drains into the circumflex veins.

These veins receive venous blood from the corpus spongiosum on the ventral aspect of the penis and wrap around the penis to drain into the deep dorsal vein.

The superficial dorsal vein drains the penile skin and prepuce before draining via the superficial external pudendal vein into the external pudendal veins.

The deep dorsal vein further drains blood from the glans penis and corpora cavernosa before joining the prostatic venous plexus.

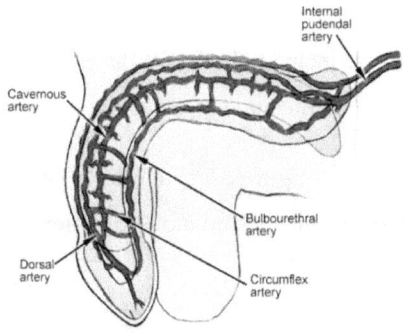

Arterial Supply of the Penis

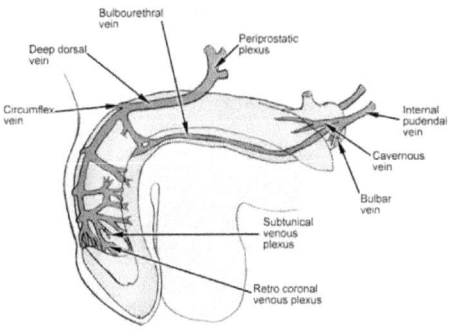

Venous Drainage of the Penis

The lymphatic drainage of the penis encompasses three locations:

– The superficial inguinal nodes (penile skin).

– Deep inguinal and external iliac nodes (glans penis).

– Internal iliac nodes (erectile tissue and urethra).

Sensory innervation to the penile skin is through the dorsal nerve of the penis, one of the terminal branches of the pudendal nerve.

Autonomic innervation includes both sympathetic and parasympathetic aspects to the corpora cavernosum via the cavernous nerves.

The sympathetic fibers originate at the level of T11-T12 and the parasympathetic fibers originate from the pelvic plexus at S2-S4.

Microscopic Anatomy

The erectile bodies of the penis are composed of fibroelastic connective tissue, smooth muscle and a network of vascular sinuses lined with endothelium.

The sinuses are continuous with the arteries that supply them and the veins that drain them.

ERECTION AND EJACULATION

In the relaxed state, the central arteries in the cavernosa are constricted, limiting blood inflow; blood flows through sinusoids, and out through veins.

In the aroused state, impulses from the brain and local nerves cause the central arteries to dilate and the muscles of the corpora cavernosa to relax.

The blood fills the sinusoids to compress the veins, reducing venous outflow and causing an erection.

As the tunica albuginea expands it compresses exiting veins to help trap blood in the corpora cavernosa, thereby sustaining the erection.

Emission is a sympathetic and parasympathetic (S2-S4) event causing peristaltic waves up the vas deferens and contractions from the seminal vesicles and prostate gland to expel contents to the prostatic urethra.

Ejaculation is expulsion of the semen in the prostatic urethra distally down the urethra.

Ejaculation occurs by expulsion of the contents of the bulbourethral glands, followed by the fluid from the epididymis and prostate, accounting for about 30% of volume and the highest sperm concentration.

Lastly, the seminal vesicles empty and produce the largest portion of the seminal volume.

Semen is an admixture of sperm cells and secretions from the male accessory sex glands that combine at the time of ejaculation.

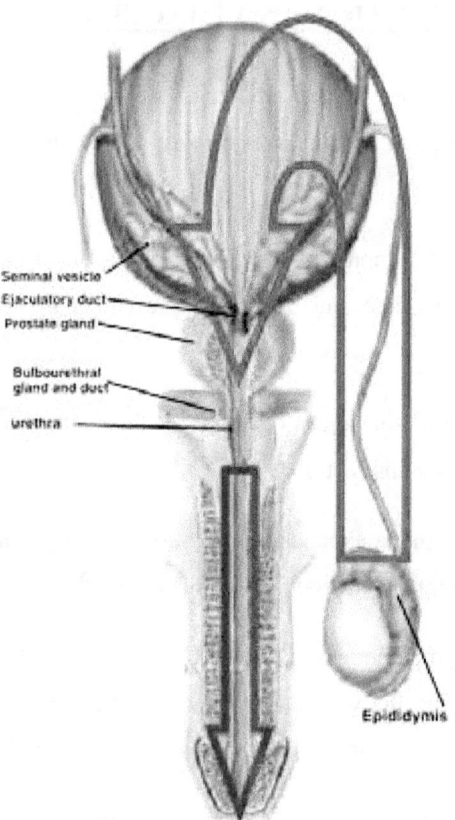

Seminal vesicle
Ejaculatory duct
Prostate gland
Bulbourethral
gland and duct
urethra

Epididymis

Mechanism of Ejaculation

POSTTESTICULAR CAUSES OF INFERTILITY

Posttesticular causes of infertility include problems with sperm transportation through the ductal system, either congenital or acquired.

Genital duct obstruction is a potentially curable cause of infertility and is observed in 7% of infertile patients.

Additionally, the sperm may be unable to cross the cervical mucus or may have ultrastructural abnormalities.

Congenital Blockage of the Ductal System

An increased rate of duct obstruction is observed in children of mothers who were exposed to DES during pregnancy.

Segmental dysplasia is defined as a vas deferens with at least 2 distinct sites of vasal obstruction.

Congenital Bilateral Absence of the Vas Deferens (CBAVD)

In congenital bilateral absence of the vas deferens, or CBAVD, the vas deferens does not develop.

Many men with CBAVD also lack much of the epididymis.

This means sperm cannot pass from the testis into the ejaculate.

However, there is normal testicular function.

Congenital bilateral absence of the vas deferens is caused by a mutation in the CFTR (cystic fibrosis transmembrane conductance regulator) gene on chromosome 7.

CFTR functions as an ion channel across the cell membrane and is the same gene involved in cystic fibrosis.

All men with cystic fibrosis have CBAVD, and 80% of men with CBAVD have documented CFTR gene mutations.

Congenital bilateral absence of the vas deferens results in obstructive azoospermia, which is non-reconstructible.

Acquired Ductal Obstruction

Acquired ductal obstruction may be due to infections in the epididymis and ejaculatory ducts or from surgery, including vasectomy, radical prostatectomy, and transurethral resection of the prostate (TURP).

Antisperm Antibodies

The blood-testis barrier is a physical barrier between the blood vessels and the maturing sperm within the seminiferous tubules of the testes.

Connections between the Sertoli cells form a tight barrier that prevents passage of cytotoxic agents into the seminiferous tubules.

Disruption of this barrier by infection, surgery, or trauma can lead to anti-sperm antibody production.

Sperm-bound antibodies can alter sperm motility and decrease fertilization ability.

Genital injury can adversely affect sperm production or sperm transport and may also lead to anti-sperm antibody production.

Scrotal surgery can inadvertently lead to ductal obstruction.

Retroperitoneal surgery can injure the nerves responsible for seminal emission.

In testicular torsion, there is twisting of the spermatic cord, which cuts off the blood supply to the testicle.

As a result, sperm production may be impaired and anti-sperm antibodies may form.

Infections and sexually transmitted infections can result in tissue damage and ductal obstruction.

Common infections include orchitis (bacterial, or secondary to mumps), epididymitis (may be due to chlamydia or bacterial) and prostatitis.

Ejaculatory Duct Obstruction

Ejaculatory duct obstruction can be congenital or acquired.

Congenital duct obstruction is due to compression and obstruction of the ejaculatory ducts by cysts within the prostate, such as müllerian duct cysts or ejaculatory duct cysts.

Acquired obstruction may be due to infections such as prostatitis or epididymitis, or related to prior urethral surgery.

The obstruction can be partial with low ejaculatory volume, or complete with azoospermia.

Ejaculatory Disorders

In retrograde ejaculation, semen enters the bladder instead of passing out through the urethra during ejaculation.

Anejaculation is the term for the inability, either physical or psychogenic, to ejaculate.

Causes of ejaculatory disorders include post-surgical changes, such as after prostate surgery; neurological alterations, such as in diabetes; spinal cord injuries; and medications, such as alpha blockers for treatment of high blood pressure and some prostate conditions.

Psychological factors can cause premature ejaculation.

Erectile Dysfunction (ED)

It is the inability to achieve or maintain an erection suitable for sexual intercourse.

Development of an erection requires intact psychological, neurological and vascular mechanisms.

Physical causes of erectile dysfunction include cardiovascular disease, diabetes, neurologic disease, and hypogonadism.

Psychogenic causes include depression, anxiety, and stress.

Medications also affect ED, especially antidepressants and drugs to treat hypertension.

MALE INFERTILITY WORKUP

History

Timing of Puberty

Precocious puberty, defined as the onset of puberty before age 9 years in males, may be the sign of a serious underlying endocrinologic disorder.

Hormonally active tumors from the testicle, adrenal gland, or pituitary, along with adrenal hyperplasia, may result in early puberty.

In contrast, a delay in puberty may be caused by problems with testosterone secretion due to hypothalamic, pituitary, or testicular insufficiency or to end-organ androgen insensitivity.

Childhood Urological Disorders

Both unilateral and bilateral cryptorchidism are associated with a decrease in sperm production and semen quality, regardless of the timing of orchidopexy.

Patients with hypospadias may not place the semen at the cervical os.

Prior bladder neck procedure, such as a V-Y plasty performed at the time of ureteral reimplantation, may lead to retrograde ejaculation.

The vas deferens or the testicular blood supply may be injured or ligated at the time of inguinal surgery, hernia repair, hydrocelectomy, or varicocelectomy.

Testicular torsion and trauma may result in testicular atrophy and the production of antisperm antibodies.

Medical History

Diabetes may cause autonomic neuropathy, neurogenic impotence, and retrograde ejaculation.

Obesity alters hormonal metabolism, leading to increased peripheral conversion of testosterone to estrogen and decreased LH pulse amplitude.

Sickle cell disease may lead to sickling and, therefore, direct testicular ischemia and damage.

Chronic renal failure leads to hypogonadism and feminization.

Liver disease may result in decreased male secondary sexual characteristics, testicular atrophy, and gynecomastia due to increased estrogen levels.

Postpubertal mumps may lead to testicular atrophy.

Sexually transmitted diseases and tuberculosis can cause obstruction of the vas deferens or epididymis.

Mycoplasma fastens itself to sperm, decreasing sperm motility.

Smallpox, prostatitis, orchitis, seminal vesiculitis, and urethritis may lead to obstructive azoospermia.

Acute and Chronic Illnesses

Anesthesia, surgery, starvation, myocardial infarction, hepatic coma, head injury, stroke, respiratory failure, congestive heart failure, sepsis, and burns are associated with a suppression of gonadotropin release, possibly through an increase in dopamine and opiate levels.

Chronic medical illnesses may directly suppress sex hormone production and sperm production, leading to end-organ failure.

Respiratory Disease

Infertility and recurrent respiratory infections may be due to immotile cilia syndrome, which may be isolated or part of Kartagener syndrome (with situs inversus).

CF is associated with congenital bilateral absence of the vas deferens (CBAVD), leading to obstructive azoospermia.

Medicines

Spironolactone, cyproterone, ketoconazole, and cimetidine have antiandrogenic properties.

Tetracycline lowers testosterone levels 20%.

Nitrofurantoin depresses spermatogenesis.

Sulfasalazine leads to a reversible decrease in sperm motility and density.

Colchicine, methadone, methotrexate, phenytoin, thioridazine, and calcium channel blockers have all be associated with infertility.

Testicular Cancer

Testicular cancer is associated with impaired spermatogenic function, even before orchiectomy, with a degree of dysfunction higher than that explained by local tumor effect.

Retroperitoneal lymph node dissection (RPLND) may impair emission (of semen into the urethra) and/or cause retrograde ejaculation.

Chemotherapy, such as cyclophosphamide, mustine, and chlorambucil, severely alter the seminiferous tubules and destroy spermatogonia.

Radiation therapy may cause irreversible spermatocytes damage, although complete recovery may be possible if stem cell are not depleted.

Spinal Cord Injury

Severe spinal cord injury may lead to anejaculation.

Epididymal and testicular factors appear to play a role, although the most severe dysfunction seems to come from prostatic and seminal vesicle.

Sexual History

The frequency, timing, and methods of coitus and knowledge of the ovulatory cycle should be elicited.

Studies show that the optimal timing for intercourse is every 48 hours at mid cycle.

Family History

Congenital midline defects, cryptorchidism, and testicular atrophy in family members may be a sign of a congenital disease.

A history of CF or hypogonadism should be elicited.

Social History

Cigarette and marijuana smoking lead to a decrease in sperm density, motility, and morphology.

Alcohol produces a chronic decrease in testosterone secretion.

Examination

Testicles

The examiner should note the presence, size, and consistency of the testicles, and the testicles should be compared with each other.

Testicular atrophy may be observed in primary testicular failure, Klinefelter syndrome, endocrinopathies, postpubertal mumps, liver disease, and myotonic dystrophy.

Swelling with pain indicates orchitis, whereas nontender enlargement may be observed in testicular neoplasms, tuberculosis, and tertiary syphilis.

Epididymis

The head, body, and tail of the epididymis should be palpated and assessed for their presence bilaterally.

An enlarged indurated epididymis with a cystic component should alert the examiner to the possibility of ductal obstruction.

Tenderness may be due to epididymitis.

Vas Deferens

Evaluate the vas for its presence bilaterally and palpate along its entire length to check for defects, induration, nodularity, or swelling.

Spermatic Cord

Check patients for the presence of a varicocele, which is the most common surgically correctable cause of infertility.

Grade 1 varicocele is defined as palpable only with Valsalva, while grade 2 is palpable at standing, and grade 3 is visible at rest.

Penis

The examination should focus on the location and patency of the urethral meatus and the presence of meatal strictures.

Penile curvature and the presence of penile plaques should be noted.

Body Habitus

A eunuchoid body habitus, consisting of infantile hair distribution, poor muscle development, and a long lower body due to a delayed closure of the epiphyseal plates, may be observed in patients with endocrinological disorders.

Rectal Examination

The prostate should be of normal size and without cysts, induration, or masses.

The seminal vesicles are usually not palpable.

MALE INFERTILITY INVESTIGATIONS

Laboratory Investigations

Semen Analysis

The semen analysis is the cornerstone of the laboratory evaluation of the infertile male.

Common instructions for semen collection are: 2 to 5 days of abstinence, with masturbation or intercourse using a special collection container / condom.

If the specimen is collected at home, it should be kept at room or body temperature and analyzed within 1 hour.

The semen analysis provides information on semen volume, concentration, motility and morphology.

Methods for semen analysis and laboratory protocols are defined by the World Health Organization (WHO).

The diagnosis of azoospermia is made only after centrifugation and examination of the pellet.

Reference values for semen parameters are not the same as the minimum values required for conception.

Men with semen parameters outside the reference ranges may be fertile and, conversely, men with values in range may be infertile.

In general, the more semen parameters that are abnormal, the more likely it is that a man will be infertile.

The following are the WHO 2010 lower reference values for semen analyses:

– Ejaculate volume may range from 1.5 to 6.8 mL

– pH greater than 7.2

– Sperm concentration of 15 million/mL

– Total sperm number of 39 million per ejaculate

– Percent motility of 40%

– Normal morphology of 4%

Abnormalities of semen analyses:

– Aspermia = no semen is present

– Azoospermia = semen is present but there are no sperm in the semen

– Severe oligospermia = less than 5 million sperm/mL

– Asthenospermia = reduced sperm motility

– Teratospermia = abnormal sperm morphology

Post-ejaculatory Urinalysis

A post-ejaculatory urinalysis is indicated for men with low-volume or absent ejaculate.

This may be due to retrograde ejaculation, lack of emission, ejaculatory duct obstruction, hypogonadism, or congenital absence of the vas deferens (CBAVD).

A post-ejaculatory urinalysis should be performed in men with ejaculation volumes of less than 1 mL, normal hormone levels and normal vasa.

For a post-ejaculatory urinalysis, urine should be collected after ejaculation.

The specimen is centrifuged for 10 minutes, preferably at 3000 g., and the pellet is examined at 400x magnification.

In men with azoospermia or aspermia, any sperm in the urine suggests retrograde ejaculation.

Quantitation of White Blood Cells in Semen

Increased number of white blood cells in semen is associated with poor sperm function and motility.

Under wet-mount microscopy, immature germ cells and leukocytes appear the same and are called "round cells."

The use of cytologic and immunohistochemical staining helps distinguish between the two.

Men with pyospermia (greater than 1 million leukocytes/mL) should be evaluated for genital tract infection or inflammation.

Sperm Viability Tests

Sperm viability tests are indicated when the sperm motility is less than 5%.

These tests help determine whether non-motile sperm are viable.

Eosin Y and trypan blue dye tests identify intact cell membranes in viable sperm by the ability of the cell to exclude the stain and remain colorless.

Sperm used in this test cannot be used in IVF.

In the hypoosmotic swelling test (HOS), viable sperm with intact cell-membrane function swell when placed in a hypoosmotic solution.

Sperm from this test can be used for IVF.

Sperm DNA Fragmentation Tests

Sperm DNA fragmentation tests help determine DNA integrity, which is important for embryo development.

DNA fragmentation refers to double-stranded breaks in sperm DNA that cannot be repaired.

Sperm DNA damage is more common in infertile men and may contribute to poor reproduction in some couples.

DNA fragmentation rates can be measured by either direct or indirect testing.

At this time there is no proven role for routine use of this test in the evaluation of male infertility.

Antisperm Antibodies (ASA) Testing

ASA testing should be performed if there is isolated asthenospermia with normal sperm concentration or sperm agglutination.

ASA can be found in serum, seminal plasma, or directly bound to sperm.

These antibodies form when there is breakdown of the blood-testis barrier due to trauma, infection, surgery or testicular cancer.

Detection of sperm-bound antisperm antibodies is made by a direct immunobead-binding test.

The antisperm antibodies bound to sperm head or tail are clinically the most important.

Endocrine Evaluation

The male endocrine evaluation tests the hypothalamic-pituitary-testicular axis.

As endocrine disorders are uncommon in men with normal semen parameters, testing is indicated in men with abnormal semen parameters (sperm concentrations <10 million/mL), impaired sexual function, and clinical findings that suggest specific endocrinopathy.

The minimum initial endocrine evaluation should include serum FSH and total testosterone levels.

If the total testosterone level is low (<300 ng/mL), LH, prolactin levels and morning bioavailable testosterone levels should be obtained.

Reproductive endocrine levels may vary depending on the clinical condition.

In hypogonadotropic hypogonadism, all levels will be low except for prolactin.

Elevated FSH levels are associated with decreased spermatogenesis.

In testicular failure, FSH and LH are elevated (hypergonadotropic hypogonadism).

With a prolactin-secreting pituitary tumor, testosterone, LH, and FSH levels are low, and prolactin levels are elevated.

Genetic Screening

Genetic abnormalities may cause infertility by affecting sperm production or sperm transport.

Men with nonobstructive azoospermia and severe oligospermia (<5 million/mL) are at a higher risk than fertile men for having a genetic abnormality.

The most common genetic abnormalities that cause decreased sperm production are numeric and structural chromosomal aberrations and Y-chromosome microdeletions.

Men with obstructive azoospermia due to congenital bilateral absence of the vas deferens (CBAVD) most commonly have an abnormality of the cystic fibrosis transmembrane conductance regulator gene (CFTR).

Identifying the underlying genetic cause of infertility can play a significant role in determining treatment.

Cystic Fibrosis Gene Mutation

There is a strong association between CBAVD and CFTR gene mutations.

All men with CBAVD are assumed to have a CFTR gene mutation.

The female partner must be genetically tested to determine the risk of conceiving a child with cystic fibrosis.

Prevalence of CFTR mutations is also higher in men with azoospermia due to congenital bilateral epididymal obstruction and those with unilateral vasal agenesis.

Karyotypic Chromosome Abnormalities

Karyotypic chromosome abnormalities are identified in approximately 7% of infertile men.

The frequency increases in proportion to the sperm count.

Abnormalities are seen in less than 1% of men with normal sperm concentration, 5% of oligospermic men and in 10-15% of azoospermic men.

Sex chromosome aneuploidy (Klinefelter syndrome 47, XXY) accounts for two-thirds of the chromosomal anomalies seen in infertile men.

The prevalence of structural abnormalities of the autosomes (inversions, translocations) is also higher in infertile men.

Men with severe oligospermia or nonobstructive azoospermia should have karyotypes before IVF with intracytoplasmic sperm injection (ICSI) using their sperm.

Y-chromosome Microdeletions

Microdeletions of sections of the Y-chromosome can be found in 10-15% of men with azoospermia or severe oligospermia.

These occur in regions of the long arm of the Y-chromosome (Yq11), known as the azoospermia factor (AZF) regions, which contain genes necessary for spermatogenesis: AZFa is the proximal region, AZFb is the central region, and AZFc is the distal region of the arm.

The DAZ (deleted in azoospermia) gene is in the AZFc region.

Men with AZFc deletions may have severe oligospermia, or azoospermia with enough testicular sperm for retrieval.

Men with AZFa or AZFb deletions have azoospermia, and a poor prognosis for testicular sperm retrieval.

Sons of men with Y-chromosome microdeletions will inherit the abnormality and may be infertile.

Y-chromosome analysis should be offered to men with nonobstructive azoospermia and severe oligospermia before ICSI using their sperm.

Imaging Studies

Ultrasonography

Transrectal ultrasound is used to evaluate seminal vesicle diameter, ejaculatory duct dilation, and to assess the prostate for cysts.

It can help diagnose ejaculatory duct obstruction and may be used in men with low volume azoospermic ejaculates, palpable vasa and normal testicular size.

Scrotal ultrasound is used to identify varicoceles and epididymal dilation, and can identify testicular tumors.

Color-flow ultrasonography is used to evaluate for variocele using a 7- to 10-MHz probe.

A varicocele is diagnosed on a sonogram if a spermatic vein is greater than 3 mm or vein size increases with Valsalva.

Vasography

Vasography is used to evaluate patency of the ductal system.

Indications for vasography include azoospermia with mature spermatids present on testicular biopsy and at least one palpable vas.

Relative indications include severe oligospermia with a normal finding on testis biopsy, antisperm antibodies, and decreased semen viscosity.

This test may be performed either as an open procedure at the same time as testicular biopsy or by a percutaneous puncture.

Unilateral patency rules out vasal or ejaculatory duct obstruction as the cause of azoospermia.

Testicular Biopsy and Histology

Testicular biopsy is indicated in azoospermic men with a normal-sized testis and normal hormonal studies to evaluate for ductal obstruction, to further evaluate idiopathic infertility, and to retrieve sperm.

Primary testicular failure causes various defects.

Normal-sized seminiferous tubules, normal Leydig cells and Sertoli cells, and a normal tunica propria characterize maturation arrest, but germ cells are arrested at any premature stage.

Patients with hypospermatogenesis have a thin germinal epithelium and a decreased number of germinal elements.

Germ cell aplasia (Sertoli-cell-only syndrome) is associated with vacuolated Sertoli cells and no germinal epithelium but otherwise normal seminiferous tubules.

Klinefelter syndrome is characterized by a decreased number of spermatogonia, germ cell hypoplasia, Sertoli cell atrophy, tubular hyalinization, prominent Leydig cells, and deformed tubules.

Cryptorchid testes have small immature tubules, spermatogonia of variable size, and a hyalinized tunica propria.

Acute mumps orchitis is associated with interstitial edema, mononuclear infiltrate, and a degeneration of germinal epithelium, while recovery is characterized by tubular hyalinization and sclerosis.

Biopsy samples in patients with infertility due to pretesticular causes have atrophic cells due to a lack of gonadotropin stimuli.

Posttesticular obstruction leads to increased tubule diameter, increased thickness of the tunica propria, and a decreased number of Sertoli cells and spermatids, and sometimes sloughing of the germinal epithelium.

MEDICAL TREATMENT OF MALE INFERTILITY

Clomiphene Citrate

It is a potent anti-estrogen, and decreases the negative feedback to the hypothalamic/pituitary axis; this results in an increase in GnRH, and subsequently LH and FSH.

Testosterone is increased, as is estradiol, and in some men, sperm concentration will increase as well.

However, meta-analyses of randomized trials have failed to demonstrate an improvement in pregnancy rates with the use of clomiphene citrate in men for treatment of oligospermia.

Tamoxifen

Tamoxifen is another anti-estrogen that has a similar mechanism of action to clomiphene.

However, there is less estrogenic activity, so estradiol levels tend to be lower.

Similar to clomiphene citrate, no significant improvement in pregnancy rates have been seen in placebo-controlled trials.

Both of these drugs may be useful in men with low-normal testosterone levels.

Aromatase Inhibitors

Aromatase is the enzyme that catalyzes the conversion of testosterone to estradiol.

It is typically found in body fat; thus obese men tend to have higher circulating levels of estradiol.

Inhibition of this enzyme decreases estradiol levels, increases testosterone levels, and decreases the negative feedback from estrogen to the hypothalamic/pituitary axis.

Thus, this medication may be useful in obese men, although, no randomized trials have demonstrated an improvement in pregnancy rates.

Gonadotropins

For the treatment of hypogonadotropic hypogonadism, gonadotropin replacement using hCG, which is a LH analog, will increase the endogenous testosterone levels.

A regimen typically starts with a test dose of 1000 units of hCG given once a day subcutaneously for 5 days, followed by 500-1000 units given subcutaneously three times a week.

Once adequate testosterone levels have been achieved, FSH analog, such as hMG, is added until sperm production is noted in the semen.

The dosage is typically 75 units subcutaneously, three times a week for 3 to 6 months, until sperm appears.

The natural conception rate for these couples is quite high, and may approach 70% in the first year.

Androgen Therapy

Administration of exogenous androgens is counterproductive, as it will increase the negative feedback to the hypothalamus and pituitary glands.

This in turn will decrease gonadotropin release, thus removing stimulation for both testosterone and sperm production. In some patients, this may lead to sterility.

Infections

Most "infections" are not really infections, but a diagnosis based on the finding of "white blood cells" in the semen.

These cells often are round cells representing immature germ cells.

However, most labs cannot differentiate the two without the use of special stains.

For patients who have true symptomatic genital infections, the semen should be cultured.

The patient should be treated with the appropriate antibiotics, typically for 4-6 weeks, and then the semen should be recultured.

Antisperm Antibodies

Patients with antisperm antibody levels greater than 1:32 may respond to immunosuppression using cyclic steroids for 3-6 months.

However, patients need to be aware of the potential side effects of steroids, including avascular necrosis of the hip, weight gain, and iatrogenic Cushing syndrome.

Retrograde Ejaculation

Imipramine or alpha-sympathomimetics, such as pseudoephedrine, may help close the bladder neck to assist in antegrade ejaculation.

However, these medicines are of limited efficacy, especially in patients with a fixed abnormality such as a bladder neck abnormality occurring after a surgical procedure.

Alternatively, sperm may be recovered from voided or catheterized postejaculatory urine to be used in assisted reproductive techniques.

The urine should be alkalinized with a solution of sodium bicarbonate for optimal recovery.

More recently, the injection of collagen to the bladder neck has allowed antegrade ejaculation in a patient who had previously undergone a V-Y plasty of the bladder neck and for whom pseudoephedrine and intrauterine insemination had failed.

Erectile Dysfunction

Treatment of erectile dysfunction should be tailored to specific patient characteristics.

It is important that underlying medical conditions are ruled out.

Most men will respond to phosphodiesterase-5 (PDE) inhibitors (such as sildenafil); although one must be certain that the patient does not have contraindications to this treatment (for example, nitrate use).

For those who do not respond, the next step is injection therapy with vasoactive drugs, such as papaverine; these carry a higher risk of priapism (prolonged, painful erections), so care must be taken in patient selection.

Penile implants are expensive, although satisfaction is high.

Nutritional Supplementation

Nutritional supplements typically contain carnitine, which has been shown to be present in high levels in the epididymis and may be involved in sperm motility.

Most of these compounds utilize L-carnitine, acetyl-L-carnitine or both, often in combination with other supplements, such as anti-oxidants, various vitamins and trace minerals.

Although no randomized trials have demonstrated a significant benefit in pregnancy rates, one trial showed a subset of patients with improved sperm motility.

These supplements tend not to have many side effects, although they can be somewhat expensive.

Lifestyle Modification

Patients should be encouraged to stop smoking cigarettes and to limit environmental exposures to harmful substances and/or conditions.

Stress-relief therapy and consultation of other appropriate psychological and social professionals may be advised.

SURGICAL TREATMENT OF MALE INFERTILITY

The three main areas of surgical treatment include varicocele, corrective surgery for obstructive azoospermia, typically either vasovasostomy (VV) or vasoepididymostomy (EV), and sperm acquisition.

Varicocele

There are three surgical approaches to varicocele repair: retroperitoneal, inguinal and subinguinal

The low inguinal/subinguinal approaches are probably the most effective with the lowest rate of recurrence and hydrocele formation.

Varicocele repair is typically an outpatient surgery performed under local, regional, or general anesthesia.

Outcomes are improved using optical magnification to preserve the spermatic artery.

Because of the spermatogenic cycle, it typically takes 3 months to see improvement following repair.

However, improvement may take 6 months in some patients.

Approximately two thirds of patients will improve, with spontaneous pregnancy rates of up to 50% when there is no female factor present.

Vasectomy Reversal

More couples are choosing to undergo vasectomy reversal, and proper technique is important.

The goal is to achieve a sperm-tight anastomosis, which requires very small sutures (typically 9-0), magnification and experience in microsurgery.

The type of anastomosis used is dependent upon the findings during surgery.

Evidence of epididymal obstruction requires anastomosis of the vas deferens to the epididymis above the point of obstruction.

Predictors of success that can be used prior to surgery to help counsel couples include time from vasectomy, experience of the microsurgeon, length of the testicular vas remnant and the age of the female partner.

The value of the presence of sperm granuloma is debated, and none of these factors are completely predictive of outcome.

Although not major surgery, vasectomy reversal is a more invasive and technically challenging procedure than a vasectomy.

It is typically performed as outpatient procedure under local, regional or general anesthesia.

The use of a surgical microscope has become the standard, although the type of repair does not affect the outcome when performed by an experienced surgeon.

In any vasectomy reversal procedure, preservation of the blood supply is essential, as well as a sperm-tight anastomosis.

The quality of the fluid helps to determine whether a vasovasostomy or vasoepididymostomy is performed.

Some of the advantages of vasectomy reversal over sperm acquisition with IVF include the ability to conceive naturally and the possibility of more than one pregnancy.

In addition, it is typically less expensive (thus more cost effective) and does not involve treatment of the female partner.

Some of the downsides to vasectomy reversal include longer time to conception (typically 6-10 months following surgery) and variable success rates based on the factors listed above.

In addition, if the procedure is unsuccessful, sperm acquisition with IVF may become necessary.

Vasovasostomy

Generally, the procedure involves isolation of vasal ends, with or without delivery of the testis, taking care to preserve blood supply.

The vasal ends are brought into proximity with either vas clamps or suture, and fluid from the testicular vas is sampled.

It is necessary to utilize an operating microscope and very fine sutures due to size difference between the testicular lumen and the abdominal lumen of the vasal ends.

The outcome of vasovasostomy depends on quality of sperm in the vas.

Vasoepididymostomy

Currently, most microsurgeons would not perform a vasovasostomy if no sperm in the vas, but rather, would go into the epididymis and perform a vasoepididymostomy.

The epididymal tubule is intussuscepted into the vasal lumen, thus creating a sperm-tight closure.

This procedure is performed in men with epididymal obstruction due to vasectomy, epididymitis, scrotal trauma, or idiopathic epididymal obstruction.

Although the success rates are not as high as with vasovasostomy, they are still successful in approximately 75% of cases.

Sperm Acquisition Techniques

When a blockage is uncorrectable, such as with congenital bilateral absence of the vas deferens (CBAVD), or if the couple elects not to correct the obstruction, sperm may be surgically retrieved from the vas deferens, epididymis or testis for use with IVF.

Most studies demonstrate that there is no difference in outcome based on site of retrieval as long as the sperm are viable.

Furthermore, in the obstructed male, most centers do not report any difference in frozen vs. freshly retrieved sperm; however, this is lab-dependent.

Microsurgical Epididymal Sperm Aspiration (MESA)

There are several indications for microsurgical epididymal sperm aspiration (MESA).

Variants of CBAVD include idiopathic epididymal obstruction, unilateral absence of the vas with contralateral absence of the seminal vesicles, or bilateral seminal vesicle agenesis.

Although some men will undergo repeat vasectomy reversal (after a previous failed vasectomy reversal) with very good success, others choose to move to IVF.

Furthermore, if the obstruction is irreparable, sperm acquisition becomes necessary.

Finally, some couples prefer not to undergo vasectomy reversal and move straight to sperm acquisition with IVF.

Some centers no longer use MESA due to the cost and invasiveness.

However, there are still some labs that prefer motile epididymal sperm, so the procedure is still an option.

It is performed outpatient under local, regional or general anesthesia.

It does entail a scrotal incision in order to expose the epididymis, as well as an operating microscope to visualize the epididymal tubules.

Although MESA is more invasive than other forms of sperm acquisition, it does yield high numbers (often several million) motile sperm, although typically not enough for intrauterine insemination.

Since there are usually high numbers of sperm, any extra sperm can be cryopreserved for additional cycles.

MESA can be performed several times, and motile sperm are retrieved in 95% of cases.

MESA has fallen out of favor due to the increased invasiveness, cost and the need for microsurgical expertise and instruments, including the use of an operating microscope.

Percutaneous Epididymal Sperm Aspiration (PESA)

PESA is a less invasive option for obtaining epididymal sperm, with similar indications to microsurgical epididymal sperm aspiration.

It involves percutaneous aspiration of sperm from epididymis and must be utilized in conjunction with IVF.

Percutaneous epididymal sperm aspiration is typically performed under local anesthesia in the office or operating room.

The technique utilizes a 21- to 24-gauge butterfly needle, sperm wash media, and a syringe.

The epididymis is held, and multiple passes are made with needle while aspirating.

While the procedure does not require the use of magnification, there is a learning curve necessary before being able to successfully obtain motile sperm.

PESA has several advantages: it is a rapid, relatively easy, non-invasive with low cost and morbidity. It may be performed under local anesthesia in the office and no microsurgical expertise is required.

PESA disadvantages include the small numbers of sperm retrieved and the possibility of diminished sperm quality due to contamination by red blood cells, thus it is typically done during an IVF treatment cycle.

Furthermore, most published reports do not have the same high success rates as other forms of sperm acquisition, although this is also lab-dependent.

Testicular Sperm Extraction/Aspiration (TESE/TESA)

TESE/TESA has similar indications as for the microsurgical and percutaneous techniques, although it may also be used in nonobstructive azoospermia.

This technique is utilized more as labs have become more comfortable using testicular sperm.

TESE/TESA must be done in conjunction with IVF and ICSI.

TESE is typically considered an open biopsy.

This approach yields significant amounts of testicular tissue, although it is more invasive than TESA.

It may be most suitable for men with poor sperm production, as it allows for multiple biopsies.

TESA is a percutaneous technique.

Suction is created with the piston syringe handle.

After several passes, the needle is removed and the testis tissue is either grasped as it comes out or flushed from the tubing.

This approach will often yield enough tissue for multiple cycles and, if necessary, pathology.

Both can be performed as an outpatient under local, regional or general anesthesia, and may be performed in the office or the operating room.

Neither technique requires the use of magnification and one of two techniques may be utilized: delivery of the testis or window technique.

TESE/TESA procedure is a rapid, relatively easy, non-invasive method of sperm retrieval.

Multiple specimens can be cryopreserved for later use.

Disadvantage of TESE/TESA is that the lab must be familiar/comfortable working with testicular sperm.

TESA is not always successful, and may need to be converted to an open extraction procedure.

Microscopic Testicular Sperm Extraction (Micro-TESE)

Micro-TESE is based on the finding that tubules that contain sperm appear larger under an operating microscope than those that do not.

Therefore, it is possible to identify these tubules and remove them without removing large pieces of testicular tissue.

Because of the localized nature of sperm production in nonobstructive azoospermia, the other forms of sperm acquisition, e.g., MESA and PESA are not utilized in these patients.

ASSISTED REPRODUCTION TECHNIQUES

Artificial Insemination

Artificial insemination (AI) involves the placement of sperm directly into the cervix (intracervical insemination [ICI]) or the uterus (intrauterine insemination [IUI]).

AI is most useful for couples in whom who have very low sperm density or motility, or those who have unexplained infertility.

IUI allows the sperm to be placed past the inhospitable cervical mucus and increases the chance of natural fertilization.

This results in a 4% pregnancy rate if used alone and a pregnancy rate of 8-17% if combined with superovulation.

Patients in whom IUI has failed 3-6 times should consider proceeding to IVF.

In Vitro Fertilization (IVF)

IVF involves fertilization of the egg outside the body and reimplantation of the fertilized embryo into the woman's uterus.

Indications for IVF include previous failures with IUI and known conditions of the male or female precluding the use of less-demanding techniques.

IVF generally requires a minimum of 50,000-500,000 motile sperm.

Harvesting eggs initially involves down-regulating the woman's pituitary with a GnRH agonist and then performing ovarian hyperstimulation.

Follicular development is monitored by ultrasonographic examination and by checking serum levels of estrogen and progesterone.

When the follicles are appropriately enlarged, a transvaginal follicular aspiration is performed.

A mean of 12 eggs are typically retrieved per cycle, and they are immediately placed in an agar of fallopian-tube medium.

After an incubation period of 3-6 hours, the sperm are added to the medium using approximately 100,000 sperm per oocyte.

After 48 hours, the embryos have usually reached the 3- to 8-cell stage.

Two to 4 embryos are usually implanted in the uterus, while the remaining embryos are frozen for future use.

Pregnancy rates are 10-45%.

Risks include multiple pregnancies and hyperstimulation syndrome.

In Vitro Fertilization (IVF)

Gamete/Zygote Intrafallopian Transfer (GIFT/ZIFT)

These procedures allow the placement of semen (GIFT) or a fertilized zygote (ZIFT) directly into the fallopian tube by laparoscopy.

Success rates have been estimated to be 25-30% using these techniques.

Unfortunately, these procedures require general anesthesia and have associated risks.

Fertilization and implantation are not guaranteed, and these procedures cannot be performed in patients with fallopian tube obstruction.

GIFT and ZIFT are rarely used as a therapeutic option.

Intracytoplasmic Sperm Injection (ICSI)

ICSI involves the direct injection of a sperm into an egg under microscopy.

It is indicated in patients who have failed more conservative therapies or those with severe abnormalities including patients with sperm extracted directly from the epididymis or testicle.

Oocytes are processed with hyaluronidase to remove the cumulus mass and corona radiata.

A micropipette is used to hold the egg while a second micropipette injects the sperm.

The oocyte is positioned with the polar body at the 6-o'clock or 12-o'clock position, and the sperm is injected at the 3-o'clock position to minimize the risk of chromosomal damage in the egg.

After incubation for 48 hours, the embryos have usually reached the 3- to 8-cell stage.

Two to 4 embryos are usually implanted in the uterus, while the remaining embryos are frozen for future use.

A 59% fertilization rate and a 35% pregnancy rate with the use of ICSI was reported.

Fresh sperm and cryopreserved sperm appear to have similar success rates.

Risks include multiple pregnancies and hyperstimulation syndrome.

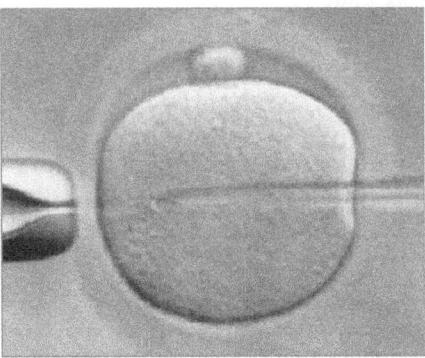

Intracytoplasmic Sperm Injection (ICSI)

MALE FERTILITY PRESERVATION

Cancer is not common in men of reproductive age; however, it is an important cause of morbidity, particularly male infertility.

As more of these cancers are cured, these men live longer and thus experience issues with infertility.

Therefore, preservation of their reproductive function is an important part of the treatment plan in these men.

Induction of infertility, as well as the degree of recovery, is due to multiple factors, including the type of treatment (chemotherapy, radiation, or surgery), the duration of treatment and the degree of injury, as well as underlying issues.

Most men who recover do so within the first 2-3 years, although it may take as long as 10 years to overcome all of these effects.

Testicular Cancer

Testicular cancer is the most common solid tumor in men of reproductive age.

Because of the advances in treatment, there is a very high cure rate (typically over 90%), so these men are now surviving and desiring fertility.

However, due to several factors, including cryptorchidism, systemic disease, disease in the contralateral testis, and endocrine abnormalities due to some of the tumor markers produced, nearly half of these men have a reduction in their baseline fertility prior to treatment.

Effects of Therapy

Radical orchiectomy, the first step in treatment, removes half of the testicular tissue.

Fortunately, most men remain fertile if no other therapy is required.

In the case of bilateral tumors or in men who have already lost a testis, partial orchiectomy is feasible if the tumor is small, localized, and the patient is willing to undergo rigorous surveillance.

Adjuvant treatment after orchiectomy, such as radiation, chemotherapy, or retroperitoneal lymph node dissection (RPLND), may further damage fertility in these men.

The nerves that control ejaculation (the sympathetic trunk) run along the aorta and can be damaged by surgery to that area.

In the case of testis cancer, this is where the lymph nodes that drain the testes lie, and the sympathetic trunk must be carefully dissected away from the lymph nodes in order to preserve ejaculatory function.

Because ejaculation is mediated by the sympathetic nervous system, injury to the sympathetic trunk can result in ejaculatory dysfunction, including anejaculation (no semen coming out) or retrograde ejaculation.

The risk of this is related to the surgical technique, as well as the type of retroperitoneal lymph node dissection performed.

The risk of ejaculatory dysfunction is nearly 100% in men undergoing this procedure after chemotherapy due to the desmoplastic response of the tumor, thus obliterating the nerves.

If a modified template (which typically spares one side of the nerves) is used for retroperitoneal lymph node dissection (without chemotherapy), the risk is still 10 to 20%.

However, if a bilateral nerve-sparing retroperitoneal lymph node dissection is performed by a surgeon skilled in this technique, the risk of ejaculatory dysfunction is less than 5%.

Preventive Measures

Preventive measures for men undergoing such procedures include banking sperm prior to any therapy and limiting radiation exposure and shielding testes during treatments.

If possible, chemotherapeutic agents with less effect on germinal epithelium should be utilized.

Patients requiring retroperitoneal surgery should be referred to experts in this area (not generalists).

Post-treatment Fertility Options

After treatment, fertility options are dependent upon whether or not there is sperm present in the ejaculate, the quality of the semen, and whether or not sperm was cryopreserved prior to treatment.

Various techniques can be performed in order to obtain sperm following testicular cancer treatment.

If the patient has retrograde ejaculation, alpha-agonists, such as pseudoephedrine, or sympathomimetics, such as imipramine, may induce antegrade ejaculation.

If retrograde ejaculation is still present, the urine may be alkalinized in order to protect the sperm and post-ejaculate urine may be collected.

If no ejaculate is present, then techniques including vibratory stimulation, electroejaculation (EEJ), vasal/epididymal/seminal vesicle aspiration and testicular sperm extraction (TESE/TESA) may be utilized.

Recommendations

All cancer patients should be directed to cryopreserve sperm prior to starting any type of cancer treatment.

Patients should also be instructed to refrain from conception for at least 6 to 12 months following radiation or chemotherapy.

Patients should be counseled about banking sperm; if they are able to provide ejaculated sample, they should do so; if unable, they should be referred for potential sperm retrieval.

Efforts should be made to minimize surgical and / or medical morbidity; shielding or dose reduction will not prevent problems; also, surgical technique matters.

Finally, microsurgery and assisted reproductive technology can overcome even severe abnormalities.

REFERENCES

– Abdel-Meguid TA, Al-Sayyad A, Tayib A, et al. Does varicocele repair improve male infertility? An evidence-based perspective from a randomized, controlled trial. Eur Urol. 2011; 59: 455-61.

– Agarwal A, Prabakaran SA, Said TM. Prevention of Oxidative Stress Injury to Sperm. Journal of Andrology. 2005; 26: 654-60.

– Al Bakri A, Lo K, Grober E, et al. Time for improvement in semen parameters after varicocelectomy. J Urol. 2012; 187: 227-31.

– Anger JT, Goldstein M. Intravasal "toothpaste" in men with obstructive azoospermia is derived from the vasal epithelium, not sperm. J Urol. 2004; 172: 634-6.

– Baccetti BM, Bruni E, Capitani S, et al. Studies on varicocele III: ultrastructural sperm evaluation and 18, X and Y aneuploidies. J Androl. 2006; 27: 94-101.

– Berookhim BM, Mulhall JP. Outcomes of operative sperm retrieval strategies for fertility preservation among males scheduled to undergo cancer treatment. Fertil Steril. 2014; 101: 805-11.

– Bhasin S, Mallidis C, Ma K. The genetic basis of infertility in men. Baillieres Best Pract Res Clin Endocrinol Metab. 2000; 14: 363-388.

– Bouloux P, Warne DW, Loumaye E; FSH Study Group in Men's Infertility. Efficacy and safety of recombinant human follicle-stimulating hormone in men with isolated hypogonadotropic hypogonadism. Fertil Steril. 2002; 77: 270-3.

– Brackett NL, Lynne CM, Aballa TC, et al. Sperm motility from the vas deferens of spinal cord injured men is higher than from the ejaculate. J Urol. 2000; 164: 712-5.

– Brugh VM, Lipshultz LI. Male factor infertility. Medical Clinics of North America. 2004; 88(2): 367-85.

– Carmignani L, Gadda F, Mancini M, et al. Detection of testicular ultrasonographic lesions in severe male infertility. J Urol. 2004; 172: 1045-7.

– Cavallini G. Male idiopathic oligoasthenoteratozoospermia. Asian Journal of Andrology. 2006; 8: 143-57.

– Chung KW. Gross Anatomy. 4th ed. Philadelphia: Lippincott Williams & Wilkins; 2000.

– Cooper TG, Noonan E, von Eckardstein S, et al. World Health Organization reference values for human semen characteristics. Hum Reprod Update. 2010; 16: 231-45.

– Cooper TG, Noonan E, Von Eckardstein S, et al. World Health Organization reference values for human semen characteristics. Human Reproduction Update. 2009; 16: 231-45.

– Costabile RA, Spevak M. Characterization of patients presenting with male factor infertility in an equal access, no cost medical system. Urology. 2001; 58: 1021-4.

– Drake RL, Vogl AW, Mitchell AWM. Gray's Anatomy for Student's. 2nd ed. Philadelphia: Churchill Livingstone Elsevier; 2010.

– Eisenberg ML, Betts P, Herder D, et al. Increased risk of cancer among azoospermic men. Fertil Steril. 2013; 100: 681-5.

– Fenig DM, Kattan MW, Mills JN, et al. Nomogram to preoperatively predict the probability of requiring epididymovasostomy during vasectomy reversal. J Urol. 2012; 187: 215-8.

– Fretz PC, Sandlow JI: Varicocele-Current concepts in pathophysiology, diagnosis and treatment. In Lipshultz LI (ed.): Urologic Clinics of North America. Philadelphia: WB Saunders; 2002.

– Gaur DS, Talekar M, Pathak VP. Effect of cigarette smoking on semen quality of infertile men. Singapore Medical Journal. 2007; 48: 119-23.

– Gillen- water JY, Grayhack JT, Howards SS, et al, editors. Adult and pediatric urology. 4th ed. London: Lippincott. Williams & Wilkins; 2002.

– Giwercman A, Petersen PM. Cancer and male infertility. Baillieres Best Pract Res Clin Endocrinol Metab. 2000; 14: 453-471.

– Hauser R, Yogev L, Amit A, et al. Severe hypospermatogenesis in cases of nonobstructive azoospermia: should we use fresh or frozen testicular spermatozoa? J Androl. 2005; 26: 772-8.

– Hauser R, Yogev L, Paz G, et al. Comparison of efficacy of two techniques for testicular sperm retrieval in nonobstructive azoospermia: multifocal testicular sperm extraction versus multifocal testicular sperm aspiration. J Androl. 2006; 27: 28-33.

– Hirsh A. Male subfertility. BMJ. 2003; 327: 669-72.

– Hsiao W, Sultan R, Lee R, Goldstein M. Increased follicle-stimulating hormone is associated with higher assisted reproduction use after vasectomy reversal. J Urol. 2011; 185: 2266-71.

– Hwang K, Walters RC, Lipshultz LI. Contemporary concepts in the evaluation and management of male infertility. Nature Reviews Urology. 2011; 8: 86-94.

– Jacobsen KD, Theodorsen L, Fossa SD. Spermatogenesis after unilateral orchiectomy for testicular cancer in patients following surveillance policy. J Urol. 2001; 165: 93-6.

– Katz VL, Lentz GM, Lobo RA, et al. Comprehensive Gynecology. 5th ed. Philadelphia: Mosby Elsevier; 2007.

– Keel BA. Within- and between-subject variation in semen parameters in infertile men and normal semen donors. Fertil Steril. 2006; 85: 128-34.

– Klemetti R, Gissler M, Sevon T, et al. Children born after assisted fertilization have an increased rate of major congenital anomalies. Fertil Steril. 2005; 84: 1300-7.

– Leibovitch I, Mor Y. The Vicious Cycling: Bicycling Related Urogenital Disorders. European Urology. 2005; 47: 277-86.

– Lipshultz LI, Rumohr JA, Bennett RC. Techniques for Vasectomy Reversal. In Sandlow JI and Nagler HN (eds.): Urologic Clinics of North America. Philadelphia: WB Saunders; 2009.

– Lombardo F, Sansone A, Romanelli F, et al. The role of antioxidant therapy in the treatment of male infertility: An overview. Asian Journal of Andrology. 2011; 13: 690-7.

– Loukas M, Colburn GL, Abrahams P, et al. Gray's Anatomy Review. Philadelphia: Churchill Livingstone Elsevier; 2010.

– Male Infertility Best Practice Policy Committee of the American Urological Association; Practice Committee of the American Society for Reproductive Medicine. Report on optimal evaluation of the infertile male. Fertil Steril. 2006; 86: S202-9.

– McCallum TJ, Milunsky JM, Cunningham DL, et al. Fertility in men with cystic fibrosis: an update on current surgical practices and outcomes. Chest. 2000; 118: 1059-62.

– Mills JN, Meacham RB. Nonsurgical Treatment of male infertility. In Lipshultz L, Howards S, and Niederberger C (eds). Infertility in the Male, 4th ed. Cambridge: Cambridge University Press; 2009.

– Neill J. Knobil and Neill's Physiology of Reproduction. 3rd ed. St. Louis, MO: Elsevier; 2006.

– Olson CK, Keppler KM, Romitti PA, et al. In vitro fertilization is associated with an increase in major birth defects. Fertil Steril. 2005; 84: 1308-15.

– Omurtag K, Cooper A, Bullock A, et al. Sperm recovery and IVF after testicular sperm extraction (TESE): effect of male diagnosis and use of off-site surgical centers on sperm recovery and IVF. PLoS One. 2013; 8: e69838.

– Ovalle WK, Nahirney PC. Netter's Essential Histology. Philadelphia: Sauders Elsevier; 2007.

– Pasqualotto FF, Sobreiro BP, Hallak J, et al. Induction of spermatogenesis in azoospermic men after varicocelectomy repair: an update. Fertil Steril. 2006; 85: 635-9.

– Practice Committee of the American Society for Reproductive Medicine. Report on management of obstructive azoospermia. Fertil Steril. 2006; 86: S259-63.

– Purohit RS, Wu DS, Shinohara K, et al. A prospective comparison of 3 diagnostic methods to evaluate ejaculatory duct obstruction. J Urol. 2004; 171: 232-5.

– Raman JD, Nobert CF, Goldstein M. Increased incidence of testicular cancer in men presenting with infertility and abnormal semen analysis. J Urol. 2005; 174: 1819-22.

– Sadler T.W. Langman's Medical Embryology. 11th ed. Baltimore, Maryland: Lippincott Williams & Wilkins; 2010.

– Safarinejad MR, Safarinejad S, Shafiei N, et al. Effects of the reduced form of coenzyme q(10) (ubiquinol) on semen parameters in men with idiopathic infertility: a double-blind, placebo controlled, randomized study. J Urol. 2012; 188: 526-31.

– Salzhauer EW, Sokol A, Glassberg KI. Paternity after adolescent varicocele repair. Pediatrics. 2004; 114: 1631-3.

– Schatte EC, Orejuela FJ, Lipshultz LI, et al. Treatment of infertility due to anejaculation in the male with electroejaculation and intracytoplasmic sperm injection. J Urol. 2000; 163: 1717-20.

– Spitz A, Kim ED, Lipshultz LI. Contemporary approach to the male infertility evaluation. Obstet Gynecol Clin North Am. 2000; 27: 487-516, v.

– Standring S. Gray's Anatomy. 40th ed. Edinburgh: Elsevier Churchill Livingstone; 2008.

– Teerds KJ, de Rooij DG, Keijer J. Functional relationship between obesity and male reproduction: from humans to animal models. Human Reproduction Update. 2011; 17: 667-83.

– Traber MG, Stevens JF. Vitamins C and E: Beneficial effects from a mechanistic perspective. Free Radical Biology and Medicine. 2011; 51: 1000-13.

– Vicdan A, Vicdan K, Günalp S, et al. Genetic aspects of human male infertility: the frequency of chromosomal abnormalities and Y chromosome microdeletions in severe male factor infertility. Eur J Obstet Gynecol Reprod Biol. 2004; 117: 49-54.

– Wald M, Ross LS, Prins GS, et al. Analysis of outcomes of cryopreserved surgically retrieved sperm for IVF/ICSI. J Androl. 2006; 27: 60-5.

– Wein AJ, ed. Campbell-Walsh Urology. 9th ed. Philadelphia, Pa: Saunders Elsevier; 2007.

– Whitten SJ, Nangia AK, Kolettis PN. Select patients with hypogonadotropic hypogonadism may respond to treatment with clomiphene citrate. Fertil Steril. 2006; 86: 1664-8.

– World Health Organization. WHO Laboratory Manual for the Examination and Processing of Human Semen. 5th Edition. Geneva, Switzerland: WHO; 2010.

– Zahalsky MP, Berman AJ, Nagler HM. Evaluating the risk of epididymal injury during hydrocelectomy and spermatocelectomy. J Urol. 2004; 171: 2291-2.

www.ingramcontent.com/pod-product-compliance
Lightning Source LLC
Chambersburg PA
CBHW061150180526
45170CB00002B/707